Possibilities

that are YOU!

Volume 11: All Things in Balance

by

Alex Bennet

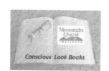

An imprint of **MQIPress** (2018)

Frost, West Virginia

ISBN 978-1-949829-09-9

MQIPress

Frost, West Virginia
303 Mountain Quest Lane, Marlinton, WV 24954
United States of America
Telephone: 304-799-7267
eMail: alex@mountainquestinstitute.com
www.mountainquestinstitute.com
www.mountainquestinn.com
www.MQIPress.com
www.Myst-Art.com

ISBN 978-1-949829-09-9
Graphics by Fleur Flohil
Opening Verse by poet Cindy Lee Scott
Cover Art by Hoi Kee Kwok

How does one balance the emotional heart
With the logical intellect mind?
Between passion and mind a harmony flow
Is not always easy to find.

For *I physically hang out in a body*
of brief temporal carnality
While I'm peering into the peculiar realm
of my spiritual reality.

Armed with the various learned lessons of self
With awareness of where I've come from;
Helps me discern the tribulations of life
And those I have yet to overcome.

Now *I physically hang out in a body*
of brief temporal carnality
While I'm peering into the peculiar realm
of my spiritual reality.

Somewhere along the way there's understanding
Of the path down which I am going;
Narrowing my focus so I can expedite
My conscious spiritual growing.

Still, *I physically hang out in a body*
of brief temporal carnality
While I'm peering into the peculiar realm
of my spiritual reality.

-Cindy Lee Scott

Preface

This book is for YOU. Regardless of economic success or educational prowess, beyond cultural influences and habitual routines, YOU have been and continue to be a student of life. And since our time in this learning sphere is precious, the challenges and opportunities are both rapid and continuous, always offering new insights. YOU are a verb, not a noun. Forget what you were taught in grammar school!

Now, we live in a world of demanding challenges, where people and systems are rebounding from control, rebelling from eras of real and perceived suppression of thought. With the acceleration of mental development over the past century has come increased awareness of human capacity, with economic success in small bites for many and large bites for the few, and for some coming with an arrogance that says, "Look at me. I'm right, you're wrong, and I'm not listening."

Because of our Economy's focus on the material, economic success begets economic success and the separation of wealth grows larger, flaming the difficulties of surviving in a CUCA world, that is, a world of accelerating change, rising uncertainty, increasing complexity, and the anxiety that comes with these phenomena.

Yet all of this **offers us, as a humanity the opportunity to make a giant leap forward.** By opening ourselves to ourselves, we are able to fully explore who we are. With that exploration comes glimmers of hope as we contemplate the power of each and every mind developed by the lived human experience!

As YOU move through your life of thoughts, feelings and actions—even when you have to repeat things over and over again as part of the experience—YOU are advancing toward the next level of consciousness.

Here's the bottom line. Everything that has been learned and continues to be learned is out there … and as a student of life, YOU have access to it all. So often it is expressed in ways that don't make sense because of the language and media being used. It just isn't presented conversationally, and you don't have a chance to ask questions from your unique point of view.

So, these little books—which we refer to as Conscious Look Books—are specifically focused on sharing key concepts from *The Profundity and Bifurcation of Change* series and **looking at what those concepts mean to YOU**.

These books are conversational in nature, and further conversations are welcome. We invite your thoughts and questions, not guaranteeing answers because there is still so much to learn, but happy to join in the conversation. Visit Mountain Quest Inn and Retreat Center www.mountainquestinn.com located in the Allegheny Mountains of West Virginia or email alex@mountainquestinstitute.com

As my partner David reminds us: *Run with the future!*

Our gratitude to all those who take this journey with us, and a special thanks to the colleagues, partners, friends, family and visitors who touch our hearts and Mountain Quest in so many ways.

With Love and Light, Alex and David

Contents

Introduction

We live in remarkable times. No doubt you've heard these words before, but there just isn't any other way to say it. Just about everywhere we look change is afoot. We are witnessing the old systems and limiting structures of the previous millennia's outdated paradigms breaking apart and crumbling around us. Major events are happening around the world in rapid sequence, including record-breaking natural disasters and unfathomable human acts the likes of which we haven't seen before. All of these are signs of change.

Many call this a time of "quickening", where the speed with which we must think, respond and take action is accelerating. Historically, change was much slower than it is today, and there was less complexity. Thus, the growth of the "normal" person was typically sufficient to maintain the balance of knowledge and action necessary to meet the change underway. Today, this is not the case. Because of the change in knowledge and action needed to effectively deal with change, it is significantly more difficult for an individual to keep up. Further, the *nature* of thinking required to meet this dynamic change—such as multi-tasking and multidimensional thinking—is significantly different because of the increasing complexity and the speed and nature of communication. *All this is preparing us for a different future*.

<<<<<<<◇>>>>>>>

INSIGHT: **Changing internal and external environments, and the nature of thinking required to meet these dynamic changes, is preparing us for a different future.**

<<<<<<<◇>>>>>>>

This idea of preparation has happened in the past. For example, following World War II, consider the number of military people provided free education in order to prepare returning veterans to find new jobs. The beginning of this shift was when women went to work in the factories, producing ten times faster than expected! Things could not fall back to the pre-war "norm". Similar shifts are occurring now. And, *the first step to dealing with an unknown future is understanding the nature of the times*.

We cannot control this. Humans often attempt to control things that are beyond their control. This can result in an imbalance, with forces pressing against you that are difficult to move through. As Allan Willis, a big picture critical thinker, describes, "The reality is that you live in a world that is uncertain and is always changing through factors that are outside of your control. The Universe is massively bigger than you are and trying to control it will have a negative impact on your balance."[1]

Human systems, which include the organizations of which we are a part, are not always in balance. Chaos theory cautions us to stay open to the unlikely, improbable and unpredictable. As business lecturer Jenifer James notes, "Chaos theory is the science of process, the knowledge of what is becoming, not what is or will remain. Our minds and our business are not always systems in balance: they are always in process."[2] Something many business people understand is that this edge of chaos can be a very creative place.

Uncertainty itself supports an interesting human trait, that is, *wrong uncertainties seem to be more satisfying than correct uncertainties*. This was understood by ancient prophets. In Hamlet's words, uncertainty "makes us rather bear those ills we have than fly to others that we know not of" (*Hamlet*, Act 3, Scene 1). This trait provides an excuse to discount an uncertain future and focus more on a known present.

[Your Thoughts]

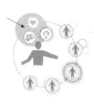

Idea 1: Every structure we see in the Universe is a result of the balancing between opposing forces of nature.

Every structure we see in the Universe is a result of the balancing between opposing forces of Nature. For example, spiral galaxies and clusters of galaxies result from a balancing between gravity and the rotation of stars as they orbit the center of the galaxy or cluster. Individual stars sustain a balance between the hydrogen gas or radiation in the center of the star pushing outwards and gravity pulling inwards. A balance occurs between gravitational and atomic forces when matter has a density close to the density of single atoms. Planets, mountains, trees, people, insects, cells, and molecules are all composed of closely packed arrays of atoms. The density of these collections of atoms is therefore similar to the density of a single one of the atoms of which they are made. Despite their superficial diversity, they are linked by a single thread—the similarity of their densities—that issues from the fact that they represent states that can withstand the crushing inward force of gravity.

Humanity can learn a great deal about balancing from Nature. Arthur Shelley, an Australian educator and businessman, determined that perhaps humans had not evolved as far as we would like to think, and that we could learn from how nature responds. As he describes: "There are many lessons that we could learn from nature, which could apply very well to the business world. The natural balance that exists in nature is something rarely achieved in human systems ... nature usually rebalances herself. It is only when humans interfere that nature loses control and falls out of balance. Could we learn from nature how to better manage our systems?"[3]

The yin and yang, ancient Chinese symbols of male and female, represent the eternally shifting balance between energies that are inseparable and contradictory opposites. This is a *Great Idea*, a timeless insight that reflects an understanding of human nature.[4] For example, take science and spirituality, once thought to be opposites but coming closer to being recognized as two different frames of reference for considering the same Universe, perhaps serving as steps toward understanding a Quantum reality.

From the balancing of opposites, wisdom can emerge. For example, psychologist Jonathan Haidt, author of *The Happiness Hypothesis*, says that a good place to look for wisdom is in the minds of your opponents, the last place you expect to find it. He reasons that you already understand the ideas common to your own side. So, if you can remove your blinders and look closely at your opponent's point of view, you may see some good ideas for the first time. This is the concept behind the Humility exercise in Idea 6 in this little book. You already know that which you know, through the richness of the diversity of others there is much more to learn! As Jonathan explains, "By drawing on wisdom that is balanced—ancient and new, Eastern and Western, even liberal and conservative—we can choose directions in life that will lead to satisfaction, happiness, and a sense of meaning. We can't simply select a destination and then walk there directly—the rider does not have that much authority. But by drawing on humanity's greatest ideas and best science, we can train the elephant, know our possibilities as well as our limits, and live wisely."[5]

Symmetry and Symbiotic Thinking

Symmetry is proportional or balanced harmony, and is tightly linked with the concept of beauty. It is the exact correspondence of form on opposite sides of a centerline or point.[6] Hermann Weyl, a mathematician, theoretical physicist and philosopher, calls symmetry a *harmony of proportions*. As he says, "Symmetry, as wide or as narrow as you may define its meaning, is one idea by which many through the ages have tried to comprehend and create order, beauty, and perfection."[7] As order, beauty and perfection, symmetry, all about balance, moves far beyond the idea of art, and is woven into the disciplines of mathematics and physics, architecture and building, and many other fields where categorization and classification are involved. The principles of symmetry penetrate every level of life.[8]

Wade says that symmetry is simultaneously a mundane and mysterious area of study. He offers that, "In itself symmetry is unlimited ... symmetry principles are characterized by a quietude, a stillness that is somehow beyond the bustling world; yet, in one way or another, they are almost always involved with transformation, or disturbance, or movement."[9]

Two common characteristics of symmetry are *congruence* and *periodicity*. Congruence refers to similar patterns and periodicity refers to regularly repeating patterns. Two different aspects of congruence are rotation and reflection. For example, a simple rotation occurs when a pattern is laid out in a circle around a central point. Symmetries abound in our everyday lives, showing up in different kinds of settings ranging from physical chemistry to classical music. For example, a butterfly's wings or the patterns in a quilt.

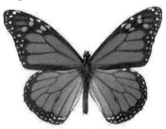

Figure 1. *An example of symmetries can be found in a butterfly's wings.*

Amazingly, four fundamental features can be used to describe any symmetrical pattern! In a book titled *The Symmetries of Things*, authors John Conway, Heidi Burgiel and Chaim Goodman-Strauss note, "It is a remarkable fact that wonders, gyrations, kaleidoscopes and mirrors suffice to describe all the symmetries of any pattern whatsoever."[10] Gyrations have repeating points around a circle; kaleidoscopes are symmetries defined by reflections; miracles occur when a pattern from one side is reflected by a pattern on the other side but does *not* go through a mirror line; and wonders are patterns that don't present the other three aspects, sort of a "catch all the rest" kind of category. Actually, maybe when you think about that last category—which sort of picks up everything that doesn't fit into the first three categories—it's not so surprising that symmetries fit into four categories!

Symmetry plays an important role in patterns and in the physical world. Nature is fond of doing things in the most economical and efficient way. As short forms of larger patterns, symbols help facilitate thinking about symmetry, and can help us recognize simpler solutions to issues and situations.

The idea of *infinite symmetry* is appealing. Actually, the idea of "infinite" anything is kind of mind-boggling! Infinite symmetry would insinuate that we know much more about the Universe than we know that we know. A popular saying in spiritual circles is, "As above, so below," which also says, "As below, so above." This means that if we can understand the models of life within our context, we have the keys to understanding higher-order patterns beyond our cognizance. While sounding like a paradox, as we discover more and more about the human mind/brain, and as we touch the thought of Quantum right here on Earth, the idea of infinite symmetry opens the doors to expanding our understanding of the Universe.

In our attempt to understand the wholeness of a topic, we are usually led to the idea of systems thinking. This extension of cause-and-effect thinking shows us that effects provide a feedback loop into the next cause. What we call an "effect" is actually *part* of the next "cause." However, through the lens of symmetry, we move from *systems* thinking to *symbiotic* thinking when we realize that the very concept of "cause" *cannot exist* without the concept of "effect." **This deeper relationship is not from causality, but from existence.**[11]

For example, would the concept of "day" exist if not also for the concept of "night?" Would we have a need for the term "summer" if not also for the term "winter?" In the physical Universe, we find that since there is such a thing as "matter," there is also "antimatter." The very existence of a thing or idea *requires* the existence of something else. We see this same pattern play out in the discussion of time and space, noting that space cannot exist without objects, and objects exist because they are surrounded by space. Does lightning just travel downward? With symbiotic thinking, we would understand that if there is a reaching down then there is also a reaching up, and indeed modern photography has captured the phenomenon of upward streamers.

As we develop our symbiotic thinking, we see that "supply and demand" is not just a single business concept, but two concepts where each exists because the other exists. We now view the old and new testaments of the Bible not as a contradiction but as a completion, since grace (new) cannot exist without law (old). And we begin to understand the nature of Quantum physics where two states must exist at the same time; for example, consider the famous thought experiment of Schrodinger's cat, which is simultaneously both alive and dead. *Things that don't make sense using systems thinking begin to make sense using symbiotic thinking.*

<<<<<<<◇>>>>>>>

INSIGHT: **Things that don't make sense using systems thinking begin to make sense using symbiotic thinking**.

<<<<<<<◇>>>>>>>

In our efforts towards co-creating the future, with symbiotic thinking there is reason to expect that our individual ideas cannot exist without also *a larger consciousness which seeks to incorporate our ideas.* The need to create cannot exist without the need to receive that which is created; and we begin to see that *there really is no creating without also co-creating.* Yet we also understand that we should expect a degree of resistance (forces) that may push against what we are creating.

Play around with this idea of symbiotic thinking. See if you can come up with some other examples. As you do this, push outside your comfort zone and have fun exploring this way of thinking! You are creating the balance of whole thinking.

Idea 2: Balanced does not mean equal.

In our search for balance, we need to first understand that **balanced does not mean equal!** Because each of us is unique with different thoughts, beliefs and feelings, *the balance of elements in which you best experience life is unique.* For example, in thinking about forces in the life experience, there are times when you *choose* to engage forces, and times when you choose to disengage. Eventually, you discover a comfortable balance that provides *the right amount of stimulation and the right amount of peace* in your personal learning journey, and you vacillate back and forth to experience the fullness of life! Yet, from a higher systems viewpoint, you are achieving balance as by choice you weigh in and out of learning experiences. An example of this is the optimum level of stress for learning and the optimum level of complexity for an organization operating as an intelligent complex adaptive system.[12]

<<<<<<<◇>>>>>>>

INSIGHT: **Balanced does not mean equal! Because you are unique with different thoughts, beliefs, feelings, etc.,** *the balance of elements in which you best experience life is unique.*

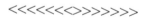

The movie *Inner World, Outer World* [13] contends that the balance of the inner and outer worlds *is the birthright of every human being*. This balance was introduced in the opening paragraphs of this little book. Balancing our inner and outer worlds is the middle way of the Buddha, and the golden mean of Aristotle. *If we can keep our life balanced, we are assisting everyone else to take a forward step.* When we are able to manage our own challenges, we become more free and independent to enjoy life, both alone and with others, and we learn to allow others the freedom to manage their challenges. When we have an inner balance, the outer world can be firing away and we are still able to function coherently. Further, there is less of an impulse to achieve balance in the exterior world when we are experiencing an inner state of balance.

<<<<<<<<>>>>>>>

INSIGHT: **When we have an inner balance, the outer world can be firing away and we are still able to function coherently.**

<<<<<<<<>>>>>>>

One approach to inner balancing is meditation. Meditation practices have the ability to quiet the conscious mind, thus allowing greater access to the unconscious.[14] In Buddhist meditation, the concept of *bare attention* is introduced to open up the mind. Bare attention is defined as "the clear and single-minded awareness of what actually happens *to* us and *in* us at the successive moments of perception."[15] The call is for us to pay attention to this very instant, the NOW, to what we are experiencing, separating our reactions from the actual events. Close your eyes for a moment and try this. It takes practice. From a Buddhist perspective, medical doctor Mark Epstein describes, "just the *bare* facts, an *exact* registering, allowing things to speak for themselves as if seen for the first time ...."[16]

More recently, Mindfulness practices are being recognized as beneficial both personally and in the workplace. Mindfulness is "a state of consciousness in which attention is focused on present-moment phenomena occurring both externally and internally."[17] This is a receptive attention, that is, the notion of meta-awareness, *being aware of being aware*. Benefits of Mindfulness include reduced stress, enhanced memory, improved focus, enhanced self-insight, and increased cognitive flexibility. There are also physiological benefits including reduced risk of cardiovascular disease.

Another approach to achieving inner balance is hemispheric synchronization, the use of sound coupled with a binaural beat to bring both hemispheres of the brain into coherence. Binaural beats were identified in 1839 by H.W. Dove, a German experimenter. In the human mind, binaural beats are detected with carrier tones (audio tones of slightly different frequencies, one to each ear) below approximately 1500 Hz.[18] The mind perceives the frequency differences of the sound coming into each ear, mixing the two sounds to produce a fluctuating rhythm and thereby creating a beat or difference frequency. Because each side of the body sends signals to the opposite hemisphere of the brain, both hemispheres must work together to "hear" the difference frequency. This perceived rhythm originates in the brainstem and is neurologically routed to the reticular formation,[19] then moving to the cortex where it can be measured as a frequency-following response.[20]

This inter-hemispheric communication is the setting for brain-wave coherence, which facilitates whole-brain cognition,[21] that is, an integration of left- and right-brain functioning.[22] What can occur during hemispheric synchronization is a physiologically reduced state of arousal while maintaining conscious awareness,[23] and, from this balanced state with both hemispheres of the brain engaged, the capacity to reach the unconscious creative state through the window of consciousness. That can be likened to being consciously awake in your sleep state.

A version of brainwave entrainment is Field Effect Audio Technology (FEAT), a trademarked product of musician and shaman Byron Metcalf,[24] that is a complex and unique integrated system of isochronic and binaural beats with specific drum and percussion rhythms and patterns. It sure makes sense that this was created by a shaman! The combined harmonics, spatial audio processing and auditory driving support a natural state of coherence and balance within us and our immediate surroundings— a phenomenon that Byron calls field effect resonance. What is fascinating about this particular product is that it builds on the drum and rattle resonances created by early man to achieve this same state. In other words, while the use of technology to assist brainwave entrainment is relatively new, the idea of creating isochronic and binaural beats for inner work has been around for thousands of years!

[Your Thoughts]

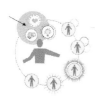

Idea 3: Self-balancing concerns important choices, starting with awareness of what is out of balance.

From the most basic perspective, the physical Universe is made up of energy and patterns of energy—nothing more, nothing less. Albert Einstein proved that everything in our material world—both animate and inanimate, organic and inorganic—*radiates* energy. The Earth and her people are an enormous energy field full of continuously flowing entangled subfields. As Jean Houston, an educator who is part of the Human Potential Movement, so aptly describes, "The Universe, we are coming to understand, is a flow that arises moment by moment from the abyss of energetic nourishment in a process of continuous regeneration."[25]

Our bodies—matter, or energy that has taken on form—are transformers of energy. The old worldview of the body as a sophisticated machine, based on Newtonian physics, is gradually giving way to a new scientific worldview of the body as a *complex energetic system*. This worldview is based on a new perspective of Quantum physics that "the biochemical molecules that make up the physical body are actually a form of vibrating energy."[26] From this new worldview, 80 percent of the etheric/dense physical plane is made up of energy;

66 percent of the astral/emotional plane is made up of energy; and 50 percent of the mental plane is made of energy.[27] In other words, regardless of whether we look from a Newtonian or Quantum viewpoint, **our everyday lives are engaged in manipulating, balancing and using energy**. We are energy beings. In a book titled *Where Ancient Wisdom and Modern Science Meet*, W. Collinge describes: "When we think of our anatomy, we ordinarily think of our bones, muscles, organs, and other physical tissues. However, we also have an *energetic* anatomy. It is composed of multiple, interacting energy fields that envelop and penetrate our physical body, govern its functioning, and extend out into the world around us. This anatomy serves as a vehicle for the circulation of vital energies that enliven and animate our lives."[28]

<<<<<<<<>>>>>>>

INSIGHT: **Our bodies—matter, or energy that has taken on form—are transformers of energy. The old worldview of the body as a sophisticated machine is gradually giving way to a new scientific worldview of the body as a complex energetic system.**

<<<<<<<<>>>>>>>

The Japanese word *Ki* describes the *essential life force*, the subtle infrastructure of our physical body, and the energy and warmth radiated by the living body, human or animal. Subtle energy is defined as low intensity vibrations/frequencies sourced from both physical (electromagnetic, Quantum, galactic) and metaphysical (consciousness, thoughts, spirit) causes. Everything that is alive contains and radiates *Ki*. Without this energetic backbone, we would have no life force and cease to exist as living, breathing, animated beings. When we open to the flow of life force, we don't have to "do" it; rather, there is an unfoldment, perhaps captured by the notion of surrendering to the flow and letting it "do" to us, fully embodying the concept of co-evolving in the NOW experience.

The free and balanced flow of *Ki* is the cause of good health.[29] Since *Ki* nourishes the organs and cells of the body, supporting them in their vital functions, the disruption of *Ki* brings about illness. In this regard, there is a direct connection between the thoughts and feelings of an individual and the flow of *Ki*. For example, *positive thoughts increase the flow of Ki and provide good feelings as well as health*. Negative thoughts disrupt the flow of *Ki* and bring about "feeling poorly".

Understanding that thoughts induce emotions and emotions affect thoughts is critical. In this continuum, there is a propensity to get caught up in a cycle of repetitive thinking where negative events just get worse and worse. This is where beliefs can come into play. A belief is a thought that you continue to think for an extended period of time. The longer you think that thought, the stronger the belief becomes, with the belief potentially influencing you to behave in a delimited manner. This paradigm explains the prejudices and opinions that limit our creativity and slow expansion of our consciousness.

As a reminder, *remember* that humans have the ability to balance their emotions. Our emotions are just that, *ours*. Although we often say, "I'm upset because of ..." or "You make me angry" or such, the emotional response we have to events and people is OURs. Once emotions are acknowledged and embraced, meeting their purpose and responsibility as a guidance system, it is our choice whether or not we continue to "feel" them. See the Conscious Little Book on *The Emoting Guidance System*.

<<<<<<◇>>>>>>

INSIGHT: **Self balancing concerns important choices. It starts with awareness of what is out of balance.**

<<<<<<◇>>>>>>

If you've been around in life for a while, you no doubt have heard the expression, and probably felt, the emotional rollercoaster of life. This is the up and down ride between excitement and disappointment, emotional highs and lows. Humans seem to have a penchant for living from one extreme to another. One approach to balance forwarded by Allan Willis is to lower your expectations as to prevent disappointment. As he says, "To free yourself from the emotional rollercoaster, have an expectation that events will be as they are going to be. Learn to accept things the way they are and do not expect events to be how you want them to be."[30]

While this is certainly one approach to achieving a "calm, relaxing and balanced journey through our lives,"[31] it also reduces the emotional feelings of vitality and being alive. Further, as we have learned from neuroscience, *our thoughts and feelings are very important to creating our reality*. Since thought form follows thought, setting intent (through expectations) is a powerful tool of self. When our thought is consistently supported by our emotions, it is like giving gas to our thought, which increases the force of our thought. There is a Conscious Look Book on *Attention and Intention*.

Emotions are a gift to humanity which, when applied well, create great harmony and connect us in Oneness. However, when mismanaged or out of balance, emotions can create conflict, negativity and war. Once we become masters of our emotional system, love and passion weave their way through all elements of our lives, guiding us toward intelligent activity and becoming the co-creators of the life we choose to live.

The equilateral triangle is often used as the basis of balancing tools. For example, two such tools are the *Lokahi* Triangle and the Life Triangle. In the

Native Hawaiian *Lokahi* tradition, balance and harmony represent the seamless unity and interconnectedness of all things. This is a reference to the concept of supernal harmony, with supernal meaning heavenly, celestial or spiritual.[32] We briefly share these below.

* * * * *

EXERCISE: *The Lokahi Triangle*

A life of harmony is one that is ordered. The *Lokahi Triangle* is an equilateral triangle with the three points representing the physical, mental and spiritual parts of a person, embedded in the environment in which they exist and entangled with a myriad of relationships, family members in the present and the past, ancestors and gods.[33] The triangle is central to the Native Hawaiian understanding of health, that the physical body cannot be healed when the triangle is out of balance, with the points working together to harmoniously participate in life.

According to Joel Levey and Michelle Levey, early pioneers in Mindfulness, these points represent nature, community and Spirit. From this viewpoint, the triangle can be used as a navigational tool, an inner compass for the journey through life. As they say, "Taking this practice to heart as a way of life cultivates a quality of continuous mindfulness regarding the vital resources that sustain your life, and encourages you to closely monitor and carefully manage the quality of relationship you have to each of these dimensions of experience."[34]

The simple wisdom of the triangle is reflected in three questions upon which the practitioner frequently pauses and reflects, assessing the truth of the responses:

REFLECTION (1): "What is the quality of my relationship to my natural world, the biosphere, and the land that sustains me?"

REFLECTION (2): "What is the quality of my relationship to my community—friends, family, colleagues—with whom I share my life?"

REFLECTION (3): "What is the quality of my relationship with Spirit, Mystery, the ground of all being, the powerful, subtle, essential dimension of all that is true and sacred?"[35]

After each question is asked, take time to reflect upon whether you are in balance with nature, community and Spirit. If the answer is yes, then reflect upon how you can deepen that relationship with balance. If the answer is no, then reflect upon how to skillfully return to a state of balance.

* * * * *

EXERCISE: *The Life Triangle*

Similarly, I've used the equilateral triangle— the *Life Triangle*—as a simple balancing tool in everyday life. The three points represent (1) physical needs, (2) relationships, and (3) personal aspirations and accomplishments. When any of the three points sinks inward and is out of balance there is discomfort, irritation and worry, and that point must become the focus of attention until balance is regained. With focus and effort, balance can be regained by the individual. Two points sinking inward are followed by deep depression, calling for immediate help and the assistance of a trusted other. With this simple understanding, the Life Triangle can be used as an assessment instrument, helping an individual pull away from the immediate issues, take a systems viewpoint of the current state of life and, when indicated, reach out for assistance.

* * * * *

From the physical perspective, the great balancer of the human body is the rhythm of rest. We all know that sleep is essential to life. This is the time when the body and mind cleanses and repairs itself, letting go of the tensions of the day. As Joel and Michelle describe, in deep sleep "our brain slows way down, and all the 'mental programs' that we run cease to operate, allowing us to rest in a state of pure being."[36] In our wake state, we have the choice of balance in terms of what we eat, the exercise we get and the thoughts and feelings that permeate our experiences.

The self also has the opportunity to balance the past, present and future through the expansion of truth. From the viewpoint of the present, the higher the level of truth of a concept the more we can understand the relationship of that concept to the past *and* the future. This is why the saying, "It's easier to know what you should have done after the fact," came into being. Indeed, looking back from the present and recognizing patterns of the past can provide healthy fodder for future decisions, as long as we're not stuck into patterns of repeating past mistakes! Truth creates visibility and expands consciousness and, *when truth becomes foundational in life then magic happens.*[37] The result is more balance, and we are more joyful and playful. Self truth comes into play here. Quite simply, "To achieve balance adjust your behavior and actions to always be true to who you are and be clear and consistent about your values."[38] Physicist MacFlouer also forwards that *virtue equals balance.*[39]

<<<<<<<<>>>>>>>

INSIGHT: **When truth becomes foundational in life, then magic happens.**

<<<<<<<<>>>>>>>

A balance important to our learning and growth is that of balancing our freedom, purpose and creativity with a consistency of choices (direction) and the actions we take. The U.S. Department of the Navy used the term *connected of choices*, acknowledging that decisions made at different parts or levels of the organization may appear conflictive and still be heading the organization in the same direction. This was based on an understanding of the wide diversity of people and knowledge, and the specific needs and contribution to the whole of each part of the organization. Understanding and embracing the idea of a connectedness of choices, and allowing the freedom and creativity at the point of action to achieve local goals while supporting the larger organizational purpose, represents movement toward intelligent activity. Recall that intelligent activity is defined as *a perfect state of interaction where intent, purpose, direction, values and expected outcomes are clearly understood and communicated among all parties, reflecting wisdom and achieving a higher truth.*

Balancing our potential and our actions is critical to a successful life. Our big thinker, Allan Willis, says that each individual has two main areas of potential (1) the ability to perform specific tasks, which is comparative to others, and (2) "the degree to which you have found balance and inner peace," which is the same for each individual.[40] He contends that fulfilling your potential runs hand-in-hand with your ability to think positively and always give your best. This, of course, refers to the power of intent and the power of thought.

When we are less than we can be, and aware of this, we live in a mix of failure and regret punctuated by fear. If we do not try, we cannot fail. If we do not share our capabilities, our limits will never be tested, or visible. Nor will we ever know the fullness of life that is our potential, our birthright.

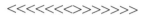

INSIGHT: **If we do not try, we cannot fail. If we do not share our capabilities, our limits will never be tested, or known.**

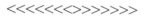

[Your Thoughts]

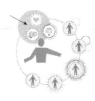

Idea 4: Balancing our outer world can be assisted by how we manage stress.

Balancing our outer world can be assisted by how we manage stress. We use the example of stress because this is a state to which almost every individual can relate as a personal example. We forward that learning is highly dependent on the level of arousal of the learner. Too little arousal and there is no motivation, too much and stress takes over and reduces learning. Thus, maximum learning occurs at the balance point where there is a moderate level of arousal.

When under stress, up to 80 percent of the blood rushes from your forebrain (the primitive brain) to your extremities and chest to support the fight-or-flight response. We lose our ability to think clearly and, instead, begin to totally "lose it." We as humans did not evolve to *think* our way out of danger. These primal behaviors were programmed into us millions of years ago when we were cave dwellers living with constant mortal danger. Thanks to the autonomic nervous system, we have automatic, rapid responses (fight, flight or freeze) that help sustain life.

As can be perceived, the body's fight-or-flight response is not intended to effectively handle the plethora of stressors that bombard us in today's modern society. For example, someone may cut you off in traffic or you may have an argument with your spouse—both of which throw you into a clear autonomic explosion of caustic stress chemicals when there is no true physical threat. Hence, our bodies react to the daily stressors of civilized life as if they were the perils of life in the Ice Age.

How can we slow or interrupt this cyclic procession of thinking, feeling and acting/behaving to allow for balance and harmony? Balancing the physiological body's stress response can serve as a key. As practiced for thousands of years, the ancient arts of yoga and Qigong accomplish energy balancing for optimal health and vitality. More recently, after studying the masters of these and other ancient arts, Donna Eden, a leader in energy medicine, established a method of self-care that consistently balanced these intermingled systems.[41] She determined that you can effectively balance your energetic body by keeping the energies *flowing in vibrant harmony* utilizing postures, movements, tapping, massaging, and holds on specific points on the skin. *Holding Neurovascular Reflect Points*, shared by Donna Panucci, a dentist and energy educator, is a simple tool that can help.

* * * * *

EXERCISE: *Holding Neurovascular Reflect Points*

Ideally, we would benefit from optimal functioning of the forebrain—the thinking part of our brain—to make prudent/wise choices under stressful circumstances. This simple yet invaluable energy technique can interrupt the stress response, as well as reprogram the way your body responds to stress.

STEP (1): Find a quiet place where you will not be caught up in the everyday sounds and movement of life for a few minutes. Close your eyes and take a few deep breaths.

STEP (2): Using your palm or fingertips, hold or touch the main Neurovascular reflect points above your eyes, with your thumbs on your temples. The Neurovascular points or frontal eminences are the raised areas on the forehead directly above the eyes. The main Neurovascular Reflex Points allow us to shift our physical body's autonomic response and assist us to meet stress with a high functioning thinking brain. They are often referred to as the "Oh my God" points, which you often intuitively hold when shocked by an alarming event. By simply holding or touching the main Neurovascular reflex points with your palm or fingertips, you boost blood and oxygen flow back up into the forebrain, allowing for clear thinking while shifting energetic patterns to calm and re-center emotionally.

STEP (3): Remaining in this position, breathe deeply for 1-5 minutes. This simple and gentle pressure instructs the primitive brain that the crisis is not a real physical threat that needs to be met with a fight-or-flight response, flooding toxic stress hormones into the bloodstream. Considering that stress reactions are physical, mental and emotional responses, this process is the foundation for reprogramming what becomes an emergency response loop.

By placing fingertips over the "Oh my God" points, thumbs on your temples and breathing deeply for 1-5 minutes while feeling stressed or focusing on a stressful memory, your mind will clear and your emotions will calm as you free yourself from your memory's emotional grip.

STEP (4): When you reach completion, thank your body for its response, take several cleansing breaths, on the out-breath releasing any tension still remaining, and open your eyes.

* * * * *

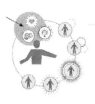

Idea 5: Balancing our senses supports the expansion of consciousness.

Without balance or senses we cannot be aware of our own consciousness. Remember that we have seven senses, the five senses of form and the additional two inner senses, which develop as we mature, emanating from the heart energy center and the crown energy center. From the heart we have a sense of connectedness with other people, a sense of Oneness. When this is coupled with feelings, it produces empathy that can lead toward compassion. This balance refers to how your learning is acted upon in service to others, the larger ecosystem of humanity, and the world at large. From the crown energy center, we have a sense of co-creating our reality as part of a larger ecosystem. When coupled with higher mental thought, we seek truth. This balance refers to the consistency of thought and feelings as we create the physical and interact with and in our creation.

We always associate seeing, hearing, smelling, tasting and touching with specific sense organs, that is, the eyes, ears, nose, mouth and hands. These senses are also connected to various energy centers within the body. While all of these energy centers work together, they are often out of balance and can become clogged with stuck energy. Let's briefly explore those energy centers—also known as chakras—and discover their relationship to our five senses of form and two internal senses.

The *root energy center*, located at the base of the spine, is associated with sexual energy and procreation, as well as our basic sense of hearing. The auditory nerve is the most complicated and connected nerve in the body. It links up with all parts of the brain, with as many as 30,000 nerve fibers at work in the inner ear alone, *making the ear the greatest supplier of sensory energy*, and the greatest changer of brain energy and direction.[42] Having 90 times greater range than our eyesight, our hearing serves as a connection to others, hearing best the sounds of other human beings around us. The ability of humans to discern the experience of others is critical to the creation of civilization and to developing a meaningful life. Of the ears, Murray Shafer, a Canadian composer, said quite succinctly, "With our eyes we are always at the edge of the world looking in, but with our ears, the world comes to us and we are always at the center of it."[43]

The *sacral energy center*, located at the base of the spine or spleen, is associated with our sense of smell, which provides a way to pick up information that is at a distance from the physical body. This energy center helps to unify and balance the energy centers, and supports inner reflection and meditation. The *solar plexus energy center*, located at the naval, is associated with the sense of touch and how we pick up information close to the physical body, allowing us to sense small degrees of change. It is also very involved in how we *emote*, that is, expressing emotion in a dramatic way. This energy center is connected to the digestive system and liver, the chemical warehouse of the body which converts energy to what is needed, allowing us to live in the physical world.

The *heart energy center*, long associated with love and the recognition of Oneness and connections, and indeed home to our internal sense of connection, allows us to love life itself, developing an understanding of life and leading to expansion of our consciousness. There is a resilience here, supporting the continuous change in which our body thrives. When we are young, there is Heart Rate Variability (HRV), that is, the distance from the peak of one heartbeat to the next varies. As we get older and become more rigid in our behaviors and thinking, the distance from the peak of one heartbeat to the next becomes more even. This regularity limits our life span; for when the heart beats in an even fashion it wears out much faster.

Heartmath, a movement to add heart to our daily activities and connections, says this resilience can be regained by establishing coherence between the heart and brain.[44] The quick methodology starts with breathing a bit slower and deeper than usual while focusing on your heart. You can tap your fingers gently in the heart area to help that focus occur. Then, think and feel positive, perhaps focusing on someone special in your life, or perhaps focusing on something for which you are extremely appreciative. It is that simple—and can be that difficult, for life is filled with past memories and current perturbations, all of which have a tendency to creep in and out of our focus.

When fully functioning, the human has the power to comprehend and empathize with others (with empathy moving into compassion), and to sense and understand the connection to a larger force, giving us an awareness beyond our own life. The energy field of the heart and the Earth's energy field are coherent, that is, *they are part of a unified field.*

* * * * *

EXERCISE: *Connecting through the Heart*

Neurons are not only located in the human brain, but in the heart, with the capability to think, feel and remember. Because these neurons are quite often not as actively engaged in everyday life as those firing within our heads, there are fewer mental models to limit the movement of our thoughts and feelings. This exercise is focused on connecting to the larger energy field through your heart.

STEP (1): Find a quiet place where you will not be bothered for a half hour. Make your body comfortable (sitting or lying down) and close your eyes.

STEP (2): Think about where your thoughts originate, and place your hand where you think that occurs. This will generally be on one side of the upper head, or on the forehead between the eyes. This "thinking spot" will serve as the starting point of your journey. Put your arm down and let your body relax.

STEP (3): Take several slow, deep breaths, breathing in through your nose and out through your mouth, consciously releasing any tensions or random thoughts with the out-breath.

STEP (4): Imagine an elevator inside the middle of your head next to the thinking spot where your thoughts originate. The door opens, and you and your thoughts enter the elevator.

STEP (5): The doors close, and you begin moving downwards. It is a beautiful elevator, see-through so you can observe yourself from within. Slowly, imagine the downward journey of the elevator, moving through the throat, down the neck, into the upper chest, and ever so slowly down right behind your heart space. Take your time; there is no hurry. Keep all of your thoughts focused from the location of your elevator. If you have difficulty imagining this slow journey, take your hand and gently trace the journey down from your thinking spot. Down, down, down, until you reach your heart space.

STEP (6): The elevator doors open and you enter your heart. It is warm, softly beating, and quite welcoming. Keeping your focus in this place, imagine yourself growing larger and larger You are energy, with no barriers. From your heart space, you expand outward, encompassing your entire body, then move beyond the body, expanding wider and wider beyond the confines of your body. You feel free, and continue expanding, wider and wider, until you fill the room or area immediately surrounding your body.

Keep your focus outward, and continue expanding, expanding, wider and wider. You, as your heart, now fill the house or field within which your body resides. Do not stop, continue expanding, periodically pausing to enjoy your growth, your freedom. Move beyond the local area to the larger geographical area of which you are a part. Keep expanding, more and more, wider and wider. You pass, and expand beyond, trees and houses, roads and the cars moving along them, up through the clouds, down into the Earth, ever-growing, expanding, expanding.

The slow rhythm of your heart gently pulses through the field. You have no limits. You become as large as the Earth, and expand beyond, reaching the limits of the solar system, and expanding even further. Continue expanding as far as you are comfortable. Then, pause and enjoy the feeling of this expansion. The lightness, yet the power of the energy of which you are a part. Observe what is beyond and, if you dare, continue expanding.

STEP (7): When you are ready to return, think about your body and where it resides, and slowly bring your awareness back to your body.

You may repeat this process any time you choose.

NOTE: After experiencing this journey, when you reflect on any issues or problems going on in your life, they may have lost their level of importance. Experiencing this journey, understanding that we are so much more, provides us with a larger systems perspective from which to view local situations.

* * * * *

The *throat energy center*, long associated with communication and providing a sense of others and how to speak to others, is also associated with our sense of taste, which is both a comparative sense and a discriminating and discerning sense. It is also connected to the lungs and breathing, and critical in controlling respiratory illnesses. The brow energy center, located between the two eyebrows, is associated with ways of seeing as well as structured energy. This is often associated with the concept of the "third eye," an inner sense of seeing. When there is too much energy flowing through this center it becomes difficult to retain our vision and use it in discriminating and discerning ways. The *crown energy center*, located at the top of the head, centers our senses themselves, connecting us to the larger Universal whole, providing a sense of morality, and opening us to discover our purpose and role in this larger whole, that is, our role as co-creators.

Development of lower mental thinking is stimulated by development of the senses. *Intelligent interaction requires senses*. For example, as you co-evolve with your environment, you get information from others and give information to others, and that information comes through your senses. If your senses are not open and well connected, then you get and give bad information. When your senses are well developed you increase the flow of information that is, in turn, used to create knowledge. In this way a balance is sustained between incoming information and action based on knowledge. This is the concept of co-evolving.

Information that leads to applied knowledge has the potential to become part of all other human beings through their senses. When this occurs, the construction of concepts (higher mental thinking) increases, and with it the level of truth also increases. This process is a *beautification of the mind*.

As an individual, **you can lighten and balance your senses**. For example, beauty has the unique capability of unifying the senses with thought, that is, capturing the attention of all of your senses with thought and feelings heading the same direction. There is a Conscious Look Book on *Transcendent Beauty*. The unification of senses with thought leads to greater levels of knowledge and creative energy, *and* expanded consciousness. Another example is the use of yoga, which is the process of joining thought and the senses of the body together, thus bringing greater balance to the senses.

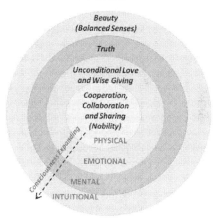

Figure 2. *Fully engaging the balanced senses on all of our planes.*

Brainwashing refers to mind control. It is the use of various techniques engaging the senses in an attempt to change the thoughts and beliefs of others against their will. In brainwashing, senses diminish such that the structure of thinking becomes discontinuous and there is a loss of sense-making ability. When the senses are not unified or balanced, there is a reduction in the ability to discern truth and untruth. Thus, brainwashing most often includes some nature of sensory deprivation or overload.

Figure 3 below represents the balancing of the physical, mental and emotional planes; the balancing of past, present and future; and the balancing of the seven senses across those planes.

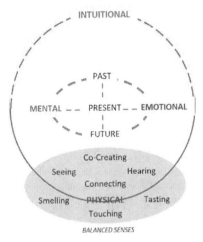

Figure 3. *The balancing of the planes, the senses and time.*

From the larger perspective of human thought, there is also the balancing of negative and positive energies. In David Hawkins' exploration of the levels of consciousness, with levels ranging from

0 to 1,000, the progression is as follows: 20 (Shame); 30 (Guilt); 50 (Apathy); 75 (Grief); 100 (Fear); 125 (Desire); 150 (Anger); 175 (Pride); 200 (Courage); 250 (Neutrality); 310 (Willingness); 350 (Acceptance); 400 (Reason); 500 (Love); 540 (Joy); 600 (Peace); and 700-1,000 (Enlightenment).[45]

It is the 200 level, the level associated with integrity and courage, that serves as a critical response point, "the balance point between weak and strong attractors, between negative and positive influence."[46] Attitudes, thoughts, feelings and associations with levels below 200 make people weaker and are associated with force; those above make people stronger and are associated with power.

Hawkin's levels of consciousness model can also be used to measure the energy of human thought. For example, David contends that only 15 percent of the populations of the world achieve the consciousness level of 200 (the critical level to move out of negativity). However, because power advances logarithmically (which follows a power law, just as earthquakes do), a single individual at the highest consciousness level (1,000, an Avatar) can "**counterbalance the negativity of all mankind**."[47] As David explains, "Were it not for these counterbalances, mankind would self-destruct out of the sheer mass of its unopposed negativity. The difference in power between a loving thought ($10^{-35 \text{ million}}$ microwatts) and a fearful thought (10^{-750}

million microwatts) is so enormous as to be beyond the capacity of the human imagination to easily comprehend. We can see ... that even a few loving thoughts during the course of the day more than counterbalance all of our negative thoughts."[48]

While I can't speak for you, I'm hoping in every single cell of my body that we have an Avatar here on Earth, or one in the works. With all the energy that is separating us and tearing us apart as a humanity, the horrific acts of disgruntled people, the pursuit of personal wealth to the detriment of others, and the atrocities of abuse and misuse visited on our ecology, it may just take an Avatar to save us and our planet and bring us back into balance!

[Your Thoughts]

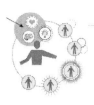

Idea 6: While we have achieved accelerated mental development, the balance of the spiritual has lagged behind.

Balance is one of the most important concepts for us to understand at this point in human history, because there are choices to make, and in many ways we are *out of balance*. Accelerated mental development and a focus on hard competition void of a spiritual counterbalance has led to expansion of the ego into arrogance, plaguing both individuals and the organizations from which we operate. While spiritual energy weaves throughout all of our planes, its balancing effects may be embraced or rejected through conscious choice.

Today, we recognize that *a balancing of our outer and inner worlds is necessary*. This important imbalance is a heme throughout this little book. As Harvey contends, we are "in a period of evolution where the world has expanded and developed outwardly and left the inner world behind. Our inner selves must catch up and restore the balance."[49] If we pause for a moment and reflect within, we can recognize the truth in this statement.

Meaning, derived from combining recognition and understanding, does not exist in the sensory or outer world. Meaning and values "are only perceived in the inner or super-material spheres of human experience."[50] It is in this inner world, which is truly creative, that advances of civilization are born. "Civilization can hardly progress when the majority of the youth of any generation devote their interests and energies to the materialistic pursuits of the sensory or outer world."[51] It is not surprising that the set of values is quite different for the inner and outer worlds. A better and more enduring civilization can only be built on the higher concepts of wisdom and virtue. This cannot occur when the younger generations focus on materialism and economics, showing no interest in ethics, sociology, philosophy, the fine arts, religion, and cosmology.[52]

With the amazing expansion of technology, the growth of knowledge has been exponential. The continuous expansion of information and knowledge is viewed as a positive reinforcing feedback loop. In his introduction to systems, Kauffman[53] uses the knowledge explosion as an example of a positive reinforcing feedback loop. The continuous expansion looks something like this: there is a lightning strike that starts a fire, which is then used to cook food, which then provides light as a torch, which then is utilized in science experiments, which then turns into modern day appliances, and so forth. As Kauffman says, "The more knowledge you have, the better off your society is, and the more people it can support to spend their time looking for more knowledge"[54] AND, the more time that can be spent creating the systems that will help manage an ever-increasing information explosion! In regards to knowledge expansion, there are no visible limits to growth.

Yet balancing loops ARE needed in terms of the physical and emotional planes. The mind/brain does *not* operate in isolation. For example, we now know from neuroscience that physical health plays a significant role in the mental and physical operation of the mind/brain. Exercise increases blood flow, burning glucose as an energy source for neuron operation, and also provides oxygen to take up the toxic electrons.[55] Exercise stimulates neurogenesis, the creation of new neurons in certain locations in the brain, and exerts a protective effect on hippocampal neurons, thus heightening brain activity. The hippocampus is part of the limbic system and plays a strong role in consolidating learning and moving information from working memory to long-term memory.[56]

Exercise boosts brainpower, stimulating the proteins that keep neurons connecting with each other.[57] This is the *use it or lose it* concept that applies both to the mind and the body, both of which need to be regularly exercised. Thus, from the viewpoint of the mind/brain in terms of interaction with the health of our physical body, we now know that: (1) Physical activity increases the number (and health) of neurons; (2) Exercise increases brainpower; and (3) Choice is necessary for benefit.

As a side thought, forced exercise does not promote neurogenesis.[58]

Further, as we've forwarded throughout this text, the material brain can influence the creation, association, and exercise of the brain patterns, while at the same time these patterns can influence the architecture of the brain. What patterns are created, how many, and how often they are utilized is influenced by the physical and mental environment within which an individual lives, and the decisions and actions that individual makes and takes. As can be seen, **there is continuous interplay between the physical and mental planes**.

And we haven't brought in the emotions. When exploring emotions as a guidance system, there are several key points from neuroscience in support of that discussion, specifically, that: (1) emotions influence all incoming information; (2) emotions can increase or decrease neuronal activity; (3) the brain can generate molecules of emotion to reinforce what is learned; (4) emotional tags influence memory recall; (5) emotions miss details but are sensitive to meaning; and (6) unconscious interpretation of a situation can influence the emotional experience.

As a reminder, Candace Pert, the author of *Molecules of Emotion*, says, "Emotional states or moods are produced by the various molecules known as neuropeptide ligands, [molecules] and what we experience as an emotion or a feeling is also a mechanism for activating a particular neuronal circuit—simultaneously throughout the brain and body—**which generates a behavior involving the whole creature**, with all the necessary physiological changes that behavior would require."[59]

Thus, there is continuous communication among the brain and the body in terms of thoughts, and the emotions connected to those thoughts. The entire body is involved in emotions, and the body drives our emotions. Thought can *directly trigger* emotions at the same time it is being *directly impacted* by our emotions!

<<<<<<<>>>>>>>

INSIGHT: **Thought can *directly trigger* emotions at the same time it is being *directly impacted* by our emotions!**

<<<<<<<>>>>>>>

Webs of Energy. Our resource physicist MacFlouer says that there are webs of energy that accumulate between our various planes, that is, between our physical and emotional planes, and between our emotional and mental planes. These webs are created from retained energy in our various senses, what we refer to as "stuck" energy, primarily related to self-centeredness and selfishness as we have focused on developing our mental faculties without a spiritual counterbalance.

To understand this concept let's consider an analogy in our physical lives, specifically, a focus on materialism. Let's say we have a passion for art, and collect beautiful paintings, which bring us great joy. Only, the passion becomes an obsession, the collection expands, and everything and everyone else takes a backseat in life. Now, we become incredibly concerned regarding theft, so we set up various protection systems, perhaps hiring people to protect this art. As various other paintings are offered for sale, we bring pressure to bear to make sure that we can obtain them, and soon we are more obsessed with acquisition and ownership than the beauty of the paintings. "I must own this!" The joy we feel moves from appreciation of beauty to appreciation of ownership, which is ego-based. Thus, selfishness of thought and feelings brings with it negative energies that separate us from the flow of life, placing burdens upon ourselves. This example involves the physical and emotional planes.

These stuck energies settle in between our various planes (see figure below), creating a web that begins with our first selfish thoughts and acts, and continues to become more intricate and heavy as we grow older and continue in this mode. These webs slow down the exchange of energy among our physical, emotional and mental senses. All of our senses bring in tiny bits of information that are then internally amplified, catalogued and organized, with the personality identifying the things of interest to store initially driven by survival, pleasure and avoidance of pain, and hopefully eventually guided in terms of preference by the maturing self. The webs of retained energy act as a force, shutting down part of our sensing capability, limiting connections and reducing consciousness. Interestingly, this is not necessarily negative as we progress through life.

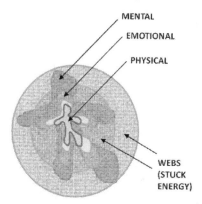

Figure 20-2. *Webs of stuck energy accumulate between the physical and emotional planes, and between the emotional and mental planes.*

How can this be valuable? Forces offer opportunities for growth and expansion. As an example, consider a time when you needed to make a decision and there were many options available and a plethora of information bombarding you that had to be taken into consideration. It's quite easy to become overwhelmed in this environment. In slowing down the processing of incoming information among our senses, we have more time to reflect on issues at hand and, hopefully, through this reflection we choose to reduce our selfishness and make decisions and take actions that are geared toward the greater good, benefiting ourselves and others. Thus, the very web we have created through selfish thoughts and feelings can provide us the opportunity to reduce our selfishness and, as this continues to occur, the web eventually ceases to exist.

As a second example, consider the web between the emotional and mental planes, that is, slowing down the processing of incoming information among the senses with an emotional and mental focus. This means that our emotions cannot immediately control our mental thought, that is, our creative imagination does not trump our mental thinking, which can happen in highly charged events. As forwarded throughout these little books, emotions are designed to support mental thought, to be used as a guidance system, not as a controlling mechanism. When the mental faculties of self are well developed, and as our consciousness expands, this web is no longer necessary. As an aside, neither are emotions intended to trump the physical senses, which are required for a coordinated response to the world around you.[60]

From this short treatment, it may be clear how important it is to achieve a balance among the mental, emotional and physical planes through which we *live our lives*, and the spiritual energy which *gives us life*. While imbalances can be useful for accelerating learning and experiencing, over a period of time imbalance can cause collapse of the system, that is, reduction of consciousness and the inability to sustain the system. Thus, **there is a finite period of time to achieve the rebalancing necessary for human sustainability**.

Yet, this balance CANNOT be achieved through over-spiritual development, which can produce fanatical or perverted interpretations of spiritual concepts. Rather, "It is to the mind of perfect poise, housed in a body of clean habits, stabilized neural energies, and balanced chemical function—when the physical, mental and spiritual powers are in triune harmony of development—that a maximum of light and truth can be imparted with a minimum of temporal danger or risk to the real welfare of such a being."[61]

The greatest barriers to learning and change are egotism and arrogance, which are fundamental difficulties in a rapidly-developing, mentally-focused business environment. Egotism says, "I am right." When egotism advances to arrogance, it says, "I am right. You are wrong. And I don't care what you think or say." As can be seen, egotism shuts the door to learning, and arrogance ceases to listen to or consider others at all, which is necessary for growth and expansion of an individual and an organization. Since others are non-existent, an arrogant individual does not care what harm is inflicted on others. Both egotism and arrogance increase the forces being produced.

Humility takes the opposite stance, opening the self to others' thoughts and ideas, and providing an opportunity for listening, reflecting, learning and expanding. Humility is the choice of letting things be new in each moment. When you remedy egotism, the self grows. Since the self is now listening to and considering others' ideas, there is larger opportunity for the bisociation of ideas, and creativity expands. Even a small amount of change can have a large impact on an individual, or humanity at large!

The simple, yet profound, conscious choice of humility can serve as a counterbalance to arrogance. Below we introduce the tool of humility, which supports openness, learning and the expansion of consciousness. This tool is borrowed from the Conscious Look Book *The Humanness of Humility.*

* * * * *

EXERCISE: *Humility*

This tool was developed from the teachings of Niles MacFlouer.[62]

STEP (1): To develop humility, first *open your mind* to accept that, by nature, at this point of development human beings have egos and desires, both of which can have strong emotional tags connected to them. It can be quite difficult for an individual to recognize egotism and arrogance in themselves. Remember, the personality, not the self, is often in control, so the individual may or may not be aware of their projection or position. This is potentially true of the individual with whom you are interacting, as well as yourself.

STEP (2): Second, *assume the other is right.* Set aside personal opinions and beliefs for the moment, accept what is being said, this idea or concept, and reflect on this new perspective in the search for truth. While this may prove quite difficult for an individual who is highly dependent on ego and arrogance to survive in what can be a challenging world, almost every individual has someone or something they love more than themselves. Try imagining that this new idea is coming from that someone or emerging from that something that you love. This simple trick will help increase your ability to engage humility.

STEP (3): Adopting this new idea or concept, *try to prove it is right*, pulling up as many examples as you can and testing the logic of it. If all the examples you can pull up fit this new perspective, then you have discovered some level of truth. If the examples contradict the concept, then bring in your ideas and test the logic of those. Again, if the examples do not all fit, continue your search for a bigger concept that conveys a higher level of truth. The critical element in this learning approach is giving up your way of thinking so that you can understand thoughts different than your own. You can compare the various concepts, asking which is more complete.

One issue that may emerge is the inclination for people to think how they feel first, then think about the logical part to determine truth. The "feeling" has already colored their higher conceptual thinking, which may result in it being untrue. It is necessary for us to develop a new sense of self that does not require us to be right in order to feel good about our thinking.

STEP (4) Once we come to a conclusion, we need to take action. It is time to affirm our incorrectness to those with whom we have potentially lacked humility, and to show gratitude for them sharing their thoughts with us. Note that the expression of appreciation and gratitude reduces forces. It is not enough to say that you were wrong, nor is that an important issue. What *is* important is to acknowledge that someone else is right, and that you are appreciative of learning from them.

STEP (5) Finally, *ensure that your motive for adopting humility is your search for truth*. Motive eventually comes out, and the wrong motive will defeat the purpose in hand. In this search for truth, you are using mental discipline to develop greater wisdom. It is difficult to overcome the urge to "look good" and to be "more right" than others. When we are "full" there is no room for new thought. When choosing humility as part of our learning journey, we discover that it is not about being right, rather it is about the continuous search for a higher truth.

* * * * *

As introduced at the beginning of this idea ... While humans have evolved, and have achieved some level of balance among the physical, emotional and mental planes that form our interactions, *the balance that the spiritual brings to all planes of existence has lagged behind.* This is largely due to the emphasis on mental development, which has escalated almost exponentially during the last decade. A considerable loss of physical capability has also accompanied this advancement of our mental faculties. Survival is no longer based primarily on the physical. Today, as a race, it would be difficult if not impossible to survive physically in the wild without technology. While survival is still a very real issue, the survival forces of today, largely based on economic worth, are headed a very different direction than those of the past. Further, since living at a survival level involves strong forces in terms of amplitude, frequency and direction, there is little energy left for being creative. For example, when you are working two jobs to put food on the table it is difficult to break out of that pattern in order to pursue your dreams. We are stuck.

What does it mean to have blocked or stuck energy? Blocked or stuck energy is in stasis, that is, a state of no change or a motionless state, often resulting from opposing forces that are balancing each other, as in our example. The force field model developed by Kurt Lewin demonstrates that a situation will stay stuck as long as there is a balance of opposing forces.[63] See the example below. *Changes can only come by upsetting this balance.*

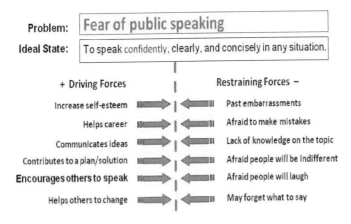

Figure xx. *A sample Force Field Analysis diagram (DON, 1999) (used with permission).*

In the figure above, ways to upset the balance would include nurturing a safe environment, gaining knowledge on the topic at hand, using well documented notes, and practicing more before speaking. As can be seen, balancing can serve as a tool to reduce forces.

One of the ways to balance opposing forces and reduce conflict is through counter-invention, that is, a *communion of opposites,*[64] which occurs naturally in change. When we invent something, we are simultaneously counter-inventing its opposite. For example, in trying to differentiate when applying for a job, an individual's education and training, which may be similar to other applicant's since it was a requirement for the job, may prevent recognition of difference. Conversely, when trying to conventionalize, the act of attaching a conventional name to something that is different may help an individual who recognizes the misfit to better perceive that difference.[65]

The bottom line is that the more successful we are at change *the greater the chance that we will end up where we began.* It is critical to understand the total process of change from a system's viewpoint in order to manage this paradoxical backlash of counter-invention and unexpected outcomes (forces). This is an interesting twist to think about!

Wow was this a long idea ... it just kept rattling out of my head. There's so much I'm still trying to understand. Hopefully, I was able to get some of these ideas out. We've so much to learn.

[Your Thoughts]

Idea 7: Dynamic balancing is required in a complex, uncertain and changing world.

Dynamic balancing is the necessary real-time balancing—symmetrization, harmonization, equalization, co-ordination and integration—of forces or demands. While *symmetrization* is used to denote a mathematical process, in a larger sense it refers to the process of making something symmetrical, a quality of having mirror images opposite each other emerging from a common center line. We introduced this earlier. *Harmonization* is bringing into harmony, bringing into agreement, adjusting differences and inconsistencies. Because I used to like to sing, I always think about it in musical terms. In music, it is the mixing of melodies and chords to create pleasing sounds.

Equalization is the act of making equal or uniform although if we think enough about it, I wonder if anything is EVER actually equal! *Co-ordination* (a "co" word, which are really important words in a global world) is having two or more elements work together effectively, efficiently and smoothly. When I think about "co" words, I like to think about people working together cooperatively and collaboratively. *Integration* is the bringing together of parts, combining them to create a whole. This is a really interesting word. In business, there are always people that are integrators, and they add so much value to the running of a business! *All of these are elements of dynamic balancing.*

Since everything is subject to change, balance in a changing, uncertain and complex environment will rarely remain constant for very long. Thus, our need in organizations for continuous learning is *actually a need for continuous learning and rebalancing*, which means (1) huge amounts of creation; and (2) a huge amount of conscious balance among these creations.[66]

When considered from the mental plane, when something is equally presented and balanced it connects to an event representing three parts of time (past, present, future). This means that it has a low degree of context sensitivity; it was true in the past, is true now and will be true in the future. For example, in a lie, at least one part of time is imbalanced; thus, something SOUNDS or FEELS untrue. Listen to this feeling. You must recognize untruths before you can respond to them. There is a Conscious Look Book on *Truth in Context*.

At the societal level, there is a balancing of freedom with the human need for security, and how much control we are willing to relinquish to the government in order to ensure that security. Examples would include the control of borders and the policing of civilians to ensure obedience in terms of laws and regulations. As musical entertainer Janis

Joplin sang many decades ago in a best-selling hit titled *Me and Bobby McGee*, "Freedom is another word for nothin' left to lose ..." Unfortunately, it is easy to push this too far. **There is a balance, and choices, that come along with advancement of society.** When this balancing of freedom, purpose and creativity does *not* happen, *energy is manifested as a substitute for intelligent activity, which then produces forces.*[67] It is then up to us to take this energy and develop higher and higher levels of intelligence.

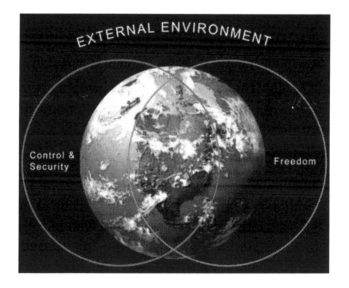

Figure 32-1. *In the words sung by Janis Joplin: "Freedom is another word for nothin' left to lose."*

Balance is not a state of being, but rather continuing, profound choices in a continuous NOW of how we interact with the world. Balancing and sensing are entangled in an interdependent relationship that actively engages us in our social environment and, if we allow it, leads to conscious compassion.

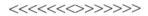

INSIGHT: **Balance is not a state of being, but rather continuing, profound choices in a continuous NOW of how we interact with the world.**

<<<<<<<<>>>>>>

As a humanity, we are bringing our consciousness back into balance as we balance development of our intellect and our deepening connections to others in pursuit of intelligent activity. However, in our acceleration of development of the mental faculties, we have focused largely on the material world and suppressed our inner spiritual senses, which can bring us into the deeper connections necessary for expansion and advancement of humanity. But no more, please. Humanity is maturing, and it is time for us to bring all that we are to the table, to reach the full potential of who we are—physical, mental, emotional and spiritual beings. It is time to bring ourselves and our world into balance.

What does this mean to me?

I sure hope I was able to convey the important issues of balance that we as individuals and as the human race are facing. You know, there's a children's book in our little shop that is titled *The Human Race*. How appropriate! I wonder if we can win that race, bringing our world into balance before we destroy it! And, what can we do to help? Hmmm. Maybe a few take-aways are a good idea.

- Changing internal and external environments, and the nature of thinking required to meet these dynamic changes, is preparing us for a different future.

- Every structure we see in the Universe is a result of the balancing between opposing forces of Nature.

- Self-balancing concerns important choices. It starts with awareness of what is out of balance.

- When truth becomes foundational in life, then magic happens.

- There is a finite period of time to achieve the rebalancing necessary for human sustainability.

- The greatest barriers to learning and change are egotism and arrogance, which are fundamental difficulties in a rapidly-developing, mentally-focused business environment.

- Balance is not a state of being, but rather continuing, profound choices in a continuous NOW of how we interact with the world.

You can see how important balance is in our lives, from cradle to death bed!

And now, as a humanity, we are called to balance an amazing mental acceleration in the outer world with a spiritual flourishing of our inner world.

It is time.

This volume of **Conscious Look Books** builds conversationally on the ideas presented in *The Profundity and Bifurcation of Change Part V: Living the Future*, largely presented in Chapter 32: "Balancing and Sensing." Co-authors of the original text include David Bennet, Arthur Shelley, Theresa Bullard, John Lewis and Donna Panucci. Full references are available in the original text, which is published by MQIPress, Frost, WV (2017), and available as an eBook on www.amazon.com

Also, excerpts from Bennet, D, Bennet, A. and Turner, R. (2015). *Expanding the Self: The Intelligent Complex Adaptive Learning System*. A New Theory of Adult Learning. Frost: MQIPress.

Endnotes

[1] Quoted from Willis, A. (2012). *Achieving Balance*. Great Britain: Manicboy Publishing, 20

[2] Quoted from James, J. (1996). *Thinking in the Future Tense: A Workout for the Mind*. New York: Touchstone, 68.

[3] Quoted from Shelley, A. (2007). *Organizational Zoo: A Survival Guide to Work Place Behavior*. Fairfield, CT: Aslan Publishing, xiii.

[4] See Haidt, J. (2006). *The Happiness Hypothesis: Finding Modern Truth in Ancient Wisdom*. New York: Basic Books.

[5] Ibid., 243.

[6] Taken from (*American Heritage Dictionary*, 2006)..

[7] Quoted from Weyl, H. (1952). *Symmetry*. Princeton, NJ: Princeton University Press, 5.

[8] See Wade, D. (2006). *Symmetry: The Ordering Principle*. New York: Walker Publishing Company.

[9] Ibid., 1.

[10] Quoted from Conway, J.H., Burgiel, H., and Goodman-Strauss, C. (2008). *The Symmetries of Things*. Boca Raton, FL: CRC Press, 27.

[11] My deep appreciation to John Lewis, a co-author of the larger work *The Profundity and Bifurcation of Change*, where this material first appeared.

[12] See Bennet, A. & Bennet, D. (2004). *Organizational Survival in the New World: The Intelligent Complex Adaptive System*. Boston, MA: Elsevier.

[13] See *Inner World, Outer World* (2012). Documentary by Daniel Schmidt. Creative Direction by Barbara Dimetto. REM Publishing Ltd. (Responsible Earth Media).

[14] See Rock, A. (2004). *The Mind at Night: The New Science of How and Why We Dream*. New York: Perseus Books Group.

[15] Quoted from Thera, N. (1962). *The Heart of Buddhist Meditation*. New York: Samuel Weiser, 30.

[16] Quoted from Epstein, M. (1995). *Thoughts Without a Thinker*. New York: BasicBooks, 110.

[17] See Dane, E. (2011) "Paying attention to mindfulness and its effects on task performance in the workplace". *Journal of Management*, Vol 37, No.4, pp 997–1018.

[18] See Oster, G. (1973). "Auditory Beats in the Brain" in *Scientific American, 229*, 94-102.

[19] See Swann, R., Bosanko, S., Cohen, R., Midgley, R., & Seed, K. M. (1982). *The Brain—A User's Manual*. New York: G.P. Putnam & Sons.

[20] See Hink, R. F., Kodera, K., Yamada, O., Kaga, K., & Suzuki, J. (1980). "Binaural Interaction of a Beating Frequency Following Responses" in *Audiology, 19*, 36-43.

[21] See Ritchey, D. (2003). *The H.I.S.S. of the A.S.P.: Understanding the Anomalously Sensitive Person*. Terra Alta, WV: Headline Books.

[22] See Carroll, G. D. (1986). *Brain Hemisphere Synchronization and Musical Learning*, reprint of paper published by University of North Carolina at Greensboro, NC.

[23] See Atwater, F. H. (2004). *The Hemi-Sync Process*. Faber, VA: The Monroe Institute. Also, Fischer, R. (1971). "A Cartography of Ecstatic and Meditative States" in *Science*, 174 (12), 897-904. Also, Delmonte, M. M. (1984). "Electrocortical Activity and Related Phenomena Associated with Meditation Practice: A Literature Review" in *International Journal of Neuroscience, 24*, 217-231. Also, Goleman, G.M. (1988). *Meditative Mind: The Varieties of Meditative Experience*. New York: G.P. Putnam. Also, Jevning, R., Wallace, R.K. & Beidenbach, M. (1992). "The Physiology of Meditation: A Review" in *Neuroscience and Behavioral Reviews, 16*, 415-424. Also, Mavromatis, A. (1991). *Hypnagogia*. Routledge, New York, NY. Also, West, M.A. (1980). "Meditation and the EEG" in *Psychological Medicine, 10*, 69-375.

[24] Taken from Metcalf, B. (2016). "Field Effect Audio Technology™ (F.E.A.T.™) FAQ" shared with author by Metcalf on 11/05/2016.

[25] Quoted from Houston, J. (2000). *Jump Time: Shaping Your Future in a World of Radical Change*. New York: Penguin Putnam Inc., 147.

[26] Quoted from Gerber, R., M.D. (2000). *Vibrational Medicine for the 21st Century. The Complete Guide to Energy Healing and Spiritual Transformation*. New York: Eagle Brook, 5.

[27] Taken from MacFlouer, Niles (2004-16). *Why Life Is...* Weekly radio shows: BBSRadio.com (#1-#480) and KXAM (#1-#143). Retrieved from http://www.agelesswisdom.com/archives_of_radio_shows.htm

[28] Quoted from Collinge, W. (1998). *Where Ancient Wisdom and Modern Science Meet ... Subtle Energy: Awakening to the Unseen forces in Our Lives*. New York: Warner Books, 20.

[29] See Rand, W. L. (1991). *Reiki: The Healing Touch*. Southfield, MI: Vision Publications, 1-9.

[30] Willis, 16.

[31] Ibid.

[32] alphaDictionary (2016). See https://www.alphadictionary.com/index.shtml

[33] See Stanford School of Medicine (2016). Ethnogeriatrics. "Traditional Health Beliefs: Native Hawaiian Values." Downloaded 09/28/2016 from https://geriatrics.stanford.edu/ethnomed/hawaiian_pacific_islander/fund/health_beliefs.html

[34] Levey, J. and Levey, M. (2014). *Living Balance: A Mindful Guide for Thriving in a Complex World*. Studio City, CA: Divine Arts, 18.

[35] Ibid., 18-19.

[36] Ibid, 125.

[37] MacFlouer (2004-16).

38 Willis, 20.

39 MacFlouer (2004-16).

40 Willis, 76.

41 See Eden, D. (2008). *Energy Medicine: Balancing Your Body's Energies for Optimal Health, Joy, and Vitality*. New York: Penguin Group.

42 See Bullard, B. and Bennet, A. (2013). *REMEMBRANCE: Pathways to Expanded Learning with Music and Metamusic®.* Frost, WV: MQIPress.

43 Quoted from Campbell, D. (2014). *Music: Physician for Times to Come.* Wheaton, Ill: Quest Books, p. 74.

44 HeartMath (2016). "The Quick Coherence® Technique". Retrieved 12/05/16 from https://www.heartmath.org/resources/heartmath-tools/quick-coherence-technique-for-adults/

45 See Hawkins, D.R. (2002). *Power VS Force: The Hidden Determinants of Human Behavior.* Carlsbad, CA: Hay House.

46 Ibid., 70.

47 Ibid., 282.

48 Hawkins, 283.

49 See Harvey, R. (2013). "The Ancient Thread of Authenticity" (An interview on Sacred Attention Therapy), 2013. Retrieved 06/13/15 from www.sacredattentiontherapy.com/Articles.html

50 *The Urantia Book* (1955). Chicago: URANTIA Foundation, 1220.

51 Ibid.

52 Ibid., 1220.

53 See Kauffman, D.L. (1980). *Systems 1: An Introduction to Systems Thinking.* Minneapolis, MN: S.A. Carlton, Publisher.

54 Ibid., 23

55 See Medina, J. (2008). *Brain Rules: 12 Principles for Surviving and Thriving at Work, Home, and School.* Seattle, WA: Pear Press.

56 Amen, D. G. (2005). *Making a Good Brain Great.* New York: Harmony Books.

57 Medina.

58 Begley, S., (2007). *Train Your Mind Change Your Brain: How a New Science Reveals Our Extraordinary Potential to Transform Ourselves.* New York: Ballantine Books.

59 Quoted from Pert, C. B. (1997). *Molecules of Emotion: A Science Behind Mind-Body Medicine*. New York: Touchstone, 145.

60 MacFlouer (2004-16).

61 Urantia, 1209.

62 Ibid.

63 See Lewin, K. (1936), *Topological Psychology*, McGraw-Hill, New York.

64 See Wagner, Roy (1975). *The Invention of Culture*. Chicago: University of Chicago.

65 McWhinney, W. (1997). *Paths of Change: Strategic Choices for Organizations and Society*. Thousand Oaks, CA: SAGE Publications, Inc., 70.

66 MacFlouer (2004-16).

67 Ibid.

The Volumes in
Possibilities that are YOU!